88 Meal and Juice Recipes to Improve Your Eye Sight:

Prevent Loss of Vision by Feeding Your Body Vitamin Rich Foods

By

Joe Correa CSN

COPYRIGHT

This publication is designed to provide accurate and authoritative information in regard to the subject matter covered. It is sold with the understanding that neither the author nor the publisher is engaged in rendering medical advice. If medical advice or assistance is needed, consult with a doctor. This book is considered a guide and should not be used in any way detrimental to your health. Consult with a physician before starting this nutritional plan to make sure it's right for you.

ACKNOWLEDGEMENTS

This book is dedicated to my friends and family that have had mild or serious illnesses so that you may find a solution and make the necessary changes in your life.

88 Meal and Juice Recipes to Improve Your Eye Sight:

Prevent Loss of Vision by Feeding Your Body Vitamin Rich Foods

By

Joe Correa CSN

CONTENTS

ABOUT THE AUTHOR

After years of Research, I honestly believe in the positive effects that proper nutrition can have over the body and mind. My knowledge and experience has helped me live healthier throughout the years and which I have shared with family and friends. The more you know about eating and drinking healthier, the sooner you will want to change your life and eating habits.

Nutrition is a key part in the process of being healthy and living longer so get started today. The first step is the most important and the most significant.

INTRODUCTION

88 Meal and Juice Recipes to Improve Your Eye Sight: Prevent Loss of Vision by Feeding Your Body Vitamin Rich Foods

By Joe Correa CSN

A proper diet is definitely a much easier way to prevent eye problems and so many other different diseases and conditions. Its influence on eye sight is often unjustly neglected because most people blame these problems with too much time on the computer or cell phone. This is true, but just like everything else, there is a lot you can do from the inside to help your body heal and strengthen on the outside. A lack of nutrients in early childhood has proven to cause eye sight problems in adulthood. This means that there is a lot you can do to help yourself and your family to prevent this problem early on.

This book contains delicious meal and juice recipes prepared with precisely chosen ingredients that will help keep your eye sight health in check. Vegetables like carrots, spinach, kale, and other leafy greens are natural antioxidants that will boost your eye nutrition and overall health.

Legumes, on the other hand, are full of precious zinc, while beans are a perfect source of bioflavonoids that prevent and lower the risk of eye health complications.

Omega-3 fatty acids can be found in fish like salmon, mackerel, and tuna. Omegas are really one of the best medicines you can possibly find in food, but when you combine them with a huge amount of vitamin A in Salmon with Carrots, you create a great combination of nutrients for your eyes.

All orange, red, and yellow vegetables are really a great source of carotenoids which is one of the best-known compounds for eye health. This is exactly why I have collected plenty of recipes based on tomatoes, sweet potatoes, carrots, and bell peppers. These recipes are healthy and tasty but at the same time will do a great job to protect your eyes.

I have used those foods to come up with tasty recipes that you can make by yourself at home. The recipes in this book offer a magnificent variety of both flavor and natural goodness, which should aid your efforts to improve the function of your eyes.

This book is a collection of meal and juice recipes that incorporate vitamins and minerals directly from Mother Nature. Zesty oranges, beneficial leafy greens, carrots, and other fruits and vegetables in various combinations will satisfy every taste. Try them all and see which ones are your favorite!

88 MEAL AND JUICE RECIPES TO IMPROVE YOUR EYE SIGHT

Meals

1. Green Pasta

Ingredients:

1 lb of broccoli, chopped

1 lb of pasta, pre-cooked

½ cup of lemon juice, freshly squeezed

2 tbsp of fresh basil, finely chopped

3 garlic cloves, minced

½ cup of almonds, roughly chopped

Preparation:

Cook the pasta using package instructions. Remove from the heat and drain well. Set aside.

Place the onions and garlic in a large nonstick frying pan over a medium-high temperature. Stir-fry for 3 minutes and then add broccoli and 1 cup of water. Cook for 10 minutes or until tender. Now, stir in pasta, lemon juice, and basil. Sprinkle some salt and pepper to taste. Add 1 more cup of water and reduce the heat. Cover with a lid and cook until liquid evaporates. Remove from the heat and top with almonds before serving.

Nutrition information per serving: Kcal: 356, Protein: 15.1g, Carbs: 58.9g, Fats: 7.4g

2. Quick Almond Pudding

Ingredients:

3/4 cup of ground almonds

1/4 cup of coconut, grated

3/4 cup of goji berries

1 cup of coconut milk

½ cup of water

1 tsp of vanilla extract

1 tsp of orange zest

1 tbsp of cornstarch

Preparation:

Combine cornstarch, vanilla extract, orange zest, and coconut milk in a deep pot. Cook for about 10-15 minutes on a low temperature. Remove from the heat and let it cool for a while.

Meanwhile, place almonds, grated coconut, goji berries and water in a food processor for 2 minutes. Add cornstarch mixture and grated coconut and mix for another 1-2 minutes.

Pour the mixture into the pudding bowls. Let it stand in the refrigerator for few hours before serving.

Nutrition information per serving: Kcal: 360, Protein: 7.1g, Carbs: 13.3g, Fats: 33.2g

3. Chicken Wings with Turmeric Sauce

Ingredients:

1lb of chicken wings, skinless

1 cup of almond milk

1 tbsp of coconut oil

2 tbsp of almond flour

1 tsp of turmeric, ground

¼ cup of olive oil

½ tsp of dried rosemary, finely chopped

¼ tsp of red pepper, ground

1 tbsp of garlic, ground

Preparation:

Preheat the oven to 300°F.

Combine rosemary, red pepper, garlic and olive oil in a large bowl. Place chicken wings coat in the marinade for about 30 minutes.

Meanwhile, melt coconut oil in a large nonstick saucepan. Add almond flour and stir for few minutes. Remove from the heat and stir in turmeric and almond milk. Return to the heat and cook for about 7-10 minutes over a medium-high temperature.

Remove the chicken wings from the marinade and place on a baking sheet. Bake uncovered for about 20 minutes. Remove from the oven, pour the turmeric sauce over the meat and bake for five more minutes. Serve with vegetables of your choice.

Nutrition information per serving: Kcal: 513, Protein: 34.8g, Carbs: 8.0g, Fats: 38.8g

4. White Beans Salad

Ingredients:

4 cups of white beans, pre-cooked

5 medium-sized onions, diced

2 cups of Romaine lettuce, chopped

2 large tomatoes, diced

2 tbsp of balsamic vinegar

2 tbsp of extra-virgin olive oil

2 medium-sized carrots, chopped

¼ cup of cilantro, chopped

2 tbsp of lemon juice

2 garlic cloves, minced

1 tsp of cumin, ground

1 tsp of sea salt

½ tsp of black pepper, ground

¼ tsp of Cayenne pepper, ground

Preparation:

Combine lemon juice, vinegar, oil, cilantro, cumin, garlic, salt, pepper, and cayenne pepper in a mixing bowl. Stir well and set aside to allow flavors to mingle.

Place the beans in a pot of boiling water. Cook until soften and remove from the heat. Drain well and transfer to a salad bowl. Stir in lettuce, tomatoes, and carrots. Drizzle with marinade and toss well to coat. Refrigerate for 10 minutes before serving.

Nutrition information per serving: Kcal: 332, Protein: 20.1g, Carbs: 57.2g, Fats: 3.7g

5. Veal Steak with Red Pepper Sauce

Ingredients:

1 lb of veal steak, boneless

3 red bell peppers, chopped

3 tbsp of olive oil

4 garlic cloves, chopped

1 small onion, peeled and chopped

1 tsp of dried rosemary, finely chopped

½ cup of water

Cooking spray

Preparation:

Preheat oven to 350°F.

Slightly coat a baking sheet with a cooking spray. Place the meat on a baking sheet and cook for 60 minutes. Remove from the oven.

Preheat the oil in a large nonstick saucepan over a medium-high temperature. Add garlic and onion and stir-fry for 5 minutes until translucent.

Add peppers, rosemary and ½ cup of water (you can add some more water if the sauce is too thick). Bring it to a boil and reduce the heat to minimum. Cook for about 10-15 minutes. Transfer to a serving plate.

Pour the pepper sauce over the meat chops and serve.

Nutrition information per serving: Kcal: 264, Protein: 24.9g, Carbs: 7.7g, Fats: 14.9g

6. Sweet Potato Tagine

Ingredients:

4 small tomatoes, chopped

1 medium-sized onion, sliced

1 medium-sized zucchini, chopped

1 cup of dry apricots

2 tbsp of olive oil

½ tsp of sea salt

2 small carrots, sliced lengthwise

2 garlic cloves, minced

2 tbsp of ginger, minced

1 tsp of cumin, ground

1 tsp of cinnamon, ground

¼ tsp of turmeric, ground

½ cup of water

2 cups of sweet potatoes, peeled and chopped into small pieces

2 tbsp of lemon juice, freshly squeezed

1 cup of canned carrots, pre-cooked and chopped

Preparation:

Preheat the olive oil in a large saucepan over a medium-high temperature. Add the onions and salt. Stir-fry for 5 minutes, or until translucent. Add carrots and fry for another 5 minutes, or until slightly soften.

Now, add the spices and raise the heat. Stir well and add tomatoes, zucchini and apricots. Pour in the water and bring it to a boil. Cover and reduce the heat. Simmer gently for about 20 minutes.

Add sweet potatoes and lemon juice. Cook uncovered until the potatoes are done and the water evaporates. Serve with a cooked carrot.

Nutrition information per serving: Kcal: 138, Protein: 2.5g, Carbs: 23.7g, Fats: 4.6g

7. Orange Carrot Smoothie

Ingredients:

2 large oranges, peeled and chopped

2 medium-sized carrots, sliced

1 cup of Greek yogurt

2 tbsp of honey

1 tbsp of flaxseeds

1 tsp of dried mint, ground

Preparation:

Combine oranges, carrots, yogurt, honey, and flaxseeds in a food processor. Blend until nicely smooth and transfer to a serving glasses. Refrigerate for 30 minutes and top with mint before serving.

Nutrition information per serving: Kcal: 155, Protein: 5.3g, Carbs: 32.0g, Fats: 1.6g

8. Baked Mushrooms in Tomato Sauce

Ingredients:

1 cup of button mushrooms, chopped

1 large tomato, diced

3 tbsp of olive oil

2 garlic, cloves

1 tbsp of fresh basil, finely chopped

½ tsp of salt

¼ tsp of black pepper, ground

Preparation:

Preheat the oven to 300°F.

Wash and peel the tomato. Cut it into small pieces. Chop garlic and mix with tomato and fresh basil.

Preheat the olive oil in a nonstick saucepan over a medium-low temperature. Add tomato and ¼ cup of water. Cook for about 15 minutes stirring constantly, or until the water evaporates. Remove from the heat.

Wash and drain mushrooms. Place them in small baking dish and spread tomato sauce over it. Add salt and pepper to taste.

Bake for about 10-15 minutes, or until doneness. Remove from the oven and serve.

Nutrition information per serving: Kcal: 205, Protein: 2.0g, Carbs: 4.9g, Fats: 21.3g

9. Cheese and Vegetable Frittata

Ingredients:

¼ cup of Cheddar cheese, crumbled

1 cup of leeks, roughly chopped

2 large tomatoes, chopped

1 cup of spinach, chopped

4 large eggs

1 small avocado, sliced

¼ cup of fresh parsley, chopped

vegetable oil spray

½ tsp of salt

¼ tsp of pepper

Preparation:

Spray some oil over a medium saucepan and preheat it to a medium-high temperature. Add leeks and cook about 4-5 minutes, or until soften. Now, add tomatoes and chopped spinach and cook for another 4-5 minutes, until all the liquid evaporates and the vegetables soften.

Meanwhile, whisk the eggs and cheese in a medium bowl. Sprinkle with salt and pour this mixture into the frying pan. Mix well with the vegetables and fry for about 3 minutes, stirring constantly.

Remove from the pan and serve with avocado slices. Sprinkle fresh parsley on top.

Nutrition information per serving: Kcal: 237, Protein: 10.5g, Carbs: 12.1g, Fats: 17.6g

10. Vanilla Rolls

Ingredients:

1 cup of almond flour

2 tbsp of coconut flour

1 tsp of baking soda

2 tsp of vanilla extract

2 tbsp of coconut oil

2 free-range eggs

¼ cup of prunes, finely chopped

¼ cup of almonds, minced

1 tsp of cinnamon, ground

Preparation:

Preheat the oven to 325°F.

Mix together almond flour, coconut flour, baking soda and vanilla extract. Add the eggs and coconut oil. Whisk together until smooth mixture. Set aside.

In another bowl, combine the prunes, minced almonds, and cinnamon. Stir well.

Transfer the dough onto a baking sheet. Roll into a long rectangle and sprinkle with the plum mixture. Cut into 7 equal pieces and let it stand in the refrigerator for about 20 minutes before baking.

Bake the rolls for about 10 minutes, or until nice golden color.

Serve warm.

Nutrition information per serving: Kcal: 160, Protein: 4.3g, Carbs: 19.0g, Fats: 7.5g

11. Buckwheat with Cranberries

Ingredients:

1 cup of fresh cranberries

1 cups of buckwheat groats

1 medium-sized apple, peeled and sliced

1 cup of Greek yogurt

3 egg whites

½ cup of maple syrup

Preparation:

Preheat the oven to 350°F.

Spread the buckwheat groats over a baking sheet and toast for about 5-6 minutes. You want a nice lightly brown color.

Boil the cranberries over a high temperature. Cook until burst. Add the toasted buckwheat groats, egg whites, apple slices, and stir well. Cook for another 7 minutes, or until the buckwheat groats are cooked. Stir in the maple syrup. Remove from the heat and let it stand for 10 minutes.

Top with yogurt and serve.

Nutrition information per serving: Kcal: 375, Protein: 12.7g, Carbs: 78.8g, Fats: 2.3g

12. Green Beans Lamb Chops

Ingredients:

2 lbs of lamb chops

2 lbs of green beans, pre-cooked

2 tbsp of fresh parsley, finely chopped

3 tbsp of olive oil

2 garlic cloves, minced

2 tbsp of rosemary, minced

½ tsp of red pepper, ground

½ tsp of salt

¼ tsp of black pepper, ground

Preparation:

Place the beans in a large nonstick skillet and pour water enough to cover all. Sprinkle with some salt and bring it to a boil. Now, cover with a lid and reduce the heat to low. Cook until soften. Remove from the heat and drain well. Transfer the beans to a large bowl, and stir in 1 tablespoon of olive oil. Toss well and set aside.

Combine parsley, garlic, red pepper, rosemary, and 1 tablespoon of oil in a large glass bowl. Place the meat in it and coat well with the mixture.

Preheat the remaining oil in a large nonstick skillet over a medium-high temperature. Cook for about 5-6 minutes on each side, or until golden brown. Remove from the heat and serve with green beans.

Nutrition information per serving: Kcal: 298, Protein: 34.1g, Carbs: 9.5g, Fats: 13.9g

13. Vegetarian Rice

Ingredients:

1 cup of couscous, uncooked

2 large carrots, sliced

½ tsp of dried rosemary, finely chopped

½ cup green olives, pitted

1 tbsp of lemon juice

1 tbsp of orange juice

1 tbsp of orange zest

4 tbsp of olive oil

½ tsp of salt

Preparation:

Wash and peel carrots. Cut into thin slices. Preheat 2 tablespoons of olive oil in a large nonstick saucepan over a medium-high temperature. Add carrots and cook for about 10-15 minutes,or until soften.Stir constantly.

Add rosemary, olives and orange juice. Mix well. Continue to cook for 3 minutes, stirring occasionally.

Combine lemon juice with 1 cup of water. Add this mixture to a saucepan and mix with remaining olive oil, orange zest and salt. Allow it to a boil and add couscous. Remove from heat and allow it to stand for about 15 minutes.

Pour these two mixtures into a large bowl and mix well with a tablespoon. Serve.

Nutrition information per serving: Kcal: 443, Protein: 8.4g, Carbs: 53.5g, Fats: 22.6g

14. Spinach Broccoli Quiche

Ingredients:

8 oz of broccoli, chopped

8 oz of spinach, chopped

1 cup of cheddar cheese, crumbled

¼ cup of heavy cream

1 cup of Mozzarella cheese, shredded

6 large eggs

1 tsp of dry mustard

1 tbsp of dill, finely chopped

½ tsp of salt

¼ tsp of black pepper, ground

Preparation:

Preheat the oven to 350°F.

Place spinach and broccoli in a pot of boiling water. Cook for 2 minutes and remove from the heat. Drain well and set aside to cool for a while.

Whisk eggs, mustard, dill, salt and pepper in a mixing bowl. Set aside.

Meanwhile, take a large baking sheet and spread the cheeses on the bottom. Make the next layer with spinach and broccoli. Pour the egg mixture on top. Place it in the oven and bake for about 25-30 minutes, or until set.

Nutrition information per serving: Kcal: 244, Protein: 17.8g, Carbs: 6.4g, Fats: 17.2g

15. Grilled Avocado in Curry Sauce

Ingredients:

1 large avocado, pitted and chopped

¼ cup of water

1 tbsp of curry powder

2 tbsp of olive oil

1 tsp of tomato sauce

1 tsp of fresh parsley, chopped

¼ tsp of red pepper, ground

¼ tsp of sea salt

Preparation:

Preheat the oil in a large saucepan over a medium-high temperature.

In a small bowl, combine curry powder, tomato sauce, chopped parsley, red pepper and sea salt. Add water and cook for about 5 minutes, stirring occasionally. Add chopped avocado, stir well and cook for another 5 minutes, or until all liquid evaporates. Turn off the heat and cover. Let it stand for about 15-20 minutes before serving.

Nutrition information per serving: Kcal: 341, Protein: 2.5g, Carbs: 11.8g, Fats: 34.1g

16. Fried Vegetables with Cottage cheese

Ingredients:

½ cup of cottage cheese

1 small onion, chopped

1 small carrot, sliced

1 small tomato, chopped

2 medium-sized bell peppers, chopped

½ tsp of salt

1 tbsp of olive oil

Preparation:

Wash and pat dry the vegetables using a kitchen paper. Cut into thin slices or strips.

Preheat the olive oil in a large saucepan over a medium-high temperature. Add the vegetables and fry for 10 minutes, stirring constantly. Add salt and mix well. You want to wait until the vegetables soften, then add soft cottage cheese. Stir well. Fry for another 2-3 minutes. Remove from the heat and serve.

Nutrition information per serving: Kcal: 121, Protein: 6.6g, Carbs: 12.4g, Fats: 5.7g

17. Creamy Leeks

Ingredients:

2 cups of leeks, trimmed

1 cup of cream cheese

½ cup of cottage cheese

1 tbsp of olive oil

½ tsp of salt

¼ tsp of black pepper, ground

A few thyme leaves

Preparation:

Cut the leeks into small pieces and wash it under cold water, a day before serving. Leave it overnight in a plastic bag.

Preheat the oil in a large nonstick skillet over a medium-high temperature. Add cottage cheese and cream cheese and fry for about 10 minutes. Add leeks, mix well and reduce the temperature to low. Fry for 10 minutes, or until soften. Remove from the saucepan and allow it to cool. Decorate with thyme leaves. Add salt and pepper to taste.

Nutrition information per serving: Kcal: 380, Protein: 11.9g, Carbs: 12.0g, Fats: 32.5g

18. Tuna with Grilled Eggplants

Ingredients:

1 lb of tuna filets, skinless and boneless

1 large eggplant, cut into bite-sized pieces

2 tbsp of balsamic vinegar

1 tbsp of lemon juice

2 tbsp of olive oil

½ tsp of salt

¼ tsp of black pepper, ground

2 tbsp of tomato sauce

1 tbsp of fresh rosemary, finely chopped

Preparation:

Preheat the grill to a medium-high temperature.

Place vinegar, tomato sauce, lemon juice, 1tablespoon of oil, salt, and pepper in a medium glass bowl. Add eggplant and coat well with marinade. Refrigerate for 10 minutes.

Preheat the remaining oil in a large nonstick skillet over a medium-high temperature. Add meat and cook for 7-10 minutes, stirring occasionally. Remove from the heat, add eggplant chops. Brush the eggplant with remaining marinade constantly. Cook until soften and serve with meat.

Add some extra salt and pepper to taste if needed.

Nutrition information per serving: Kcal: 307, Protein: 31.4g, Carbs: 7.9g, Fats: 16.5g

19. Jamaican Stew

Ingredients:

4 cups of black beans, pre-cooked

1 lb of tomatoes, diced

4 garlic cloves, minced

1 medium-sized bell pepper, chopped

1 large onion, sliced

1 tsp of curry powder

1 tsp of vegetable seasoning mix

1 tsp of thyme

1 tsp of salt

1/4 tsp of black pepper, ground

1 jalapeno pepper, minced

Preparation:

Place the beans in a pot of boiling water. Cook until soften. Remove from the heat and let it stand in water for 15 minutes.

Meanwhile, preheat the oil in a large pot over a medium-high temperature. Add onions and garlic and 2 tablespoons of water. Saute for few minutes until translucent. Now, stir in jalapeno pepper,bell pepper, thyme, curry, vegetable seasoning mix, salt, and pepper. Cook for 5 minutes, stirring occasionally.

Drain well beans and add to the pot. Pour the tomato sauce over and stir to combine. Reduce the heat to low and cover with a lid. Cook for 40 minutes and remove from the heat. Serve.

Nutrition information per serving: Kcal: 189, Protein: 22.0g, Carbs: 66.5g, Fats: 1.6g

20. Zucchini Cream Soup

Ingredients:

4 medium-sized zucchinis, chopped

3 cups of vegetable broth, unsalted

1 cup of skim milk

1 medium-sized onion, chopped

1 large bell pepper, chopped

1 tsp of dried thyme, minced

1 tbsp of vegetable oil

1 tsp of nutmeg

½ tsp of salt

¼ tsp of black pepper, ground

1 tsp of lemon zest

Preparation:

Preheat the oil in a large nonstick saucepan over a medium-high temperature. Add onions and stir-fry for 5-6 minutes, or until translucent. Add bell pepper, thyme, nutmeg, zucchini, salt, and pepper. Cook for 2 minutes more then add vegetable broth. Cook for the next 15 minutes, or until vegetables tender.

Remove from the heat and let it cool for a while. Transfer to a food processor and blend until smooth mixture. Return to the pot and add milk. Reduce the heat to low and cover with a lid. Cook for about 15-20 minutes, or until set.

Serve.

Nutrition information per serving: Kcal: 69, Protein: 4.4g, Carbs: 7.8g, Fats: 2.6g

21. Shrimp Pasta

Ingredients:

1 lb of pasta, pre-cooked

2 lb of shrimps, peeled and deveined

2 large bell peppers, chopped

5 garlic cloves, minced

4 tbsp of olive oil

¼ cup of fresh parsley, finely chopped

5 tbsp of lemon juice

1 tsp of salt

½ tsp of black pepper, ground

Preparation:

Cook the pasta using package instructions. Remove from the heat and drain well.

Preheat the oil in a large nonstick skillet over a medium-high temperature. Add shrimps and cook for 2 minutes. Add lemon juice, parsley, bell peppers and stir well. Sprinkle with some salt and pepper to taste. Cook for another 10 minutes, or until set. Remove from the heat and serve with pasta. Sprinkle with oregano and serve immediately.

Nutrition information per serving: Kcal: 374, Protein: 32.8g, Carbs: 36.0g, Fats: 10.4g

22. Asian Turkey

Ingredients:

1 lb of turkey breasts, skinless and boneless

1 tbsp of yellow mustard

1 garlic clove, minced

2 tbsp of maple syrup

1 tbsp of green tea

1 tsp of ginger, ground

1 tbsp of canola oil

½ tsp of salt

¼ tsp of black pepper, ground

Preparation:

Preheat the oven to 350°F.

Preheat the canola oil in a large nonstick saucepan over a medium-high temperature. Add garlic, ginger, maple syrup, and tea and cook for 3 minutes, stirring occasionally. Sprinkle with some salt and pepper to taste. Remove from the heat and transfer the mixture to a large bowl. Add meat and coat well with mixture. Set aside for 20 minutes to allow flavors to penetrate into the meat.

Place the meat with liquid in a large baking dish. Put it in the oven and cook for 30 minutes. Remove from the oven and peel off the skin. Serve with fresh vegetables.

Nutrition information per serving: Kcal: 361, Protein: 39.3g, Carbs: 24.7g, Fats: 11.2g

23. Avocado Lentil Salad

Ingredients:

4 cups of white lentils, pre-cooked, drain, and rinsed

1 avocado, peeled, pitted, and chopped

1 cup of lemon juice

1 medium-sized red onion, diced

2 garlic cloves, finely chopped

1 cup of fresh cilantro, finely chopped

1 tsp of chili pepper, ground

½ tsp of salt

1 tsp of lemon zest

Preparation:

Mix together lemon juice, chili pepper, salt, and lemon zest in a mixing bowl. Stir well to combine and set aside.

Place lentils in a pot of boiling water. Cook until soften and remove from the heat. Rinse with water and transfer to a large salad bowl. Add onion, garlic, and cilantro. Drizzle with marinade and toss well to combine. Top with avocado chops and before serving.

Nutrition information per serving: Kcal: 540, Protein: 34.3g, Carbs: 82.9g, Fats: 8.3g

24. Oven-Baked Shrimps and Vegges

Ingredients:

1 can of tomatoes, diced

1 can of chickpeas, drained

1 lb of shrimps, peeled and deveined

1 medium-sized onion, diced

1 cup of white rice, long-grain

2 garlic cloves, minced

1 small zucchini, chopped

3 cups of chicken stock, unsalted

2 medium-sized bell peppers, chopped

2 tbsp of olive oil

¼ tsp of salt

¼ tsp of black pepper, ground

Preparation:

Preheat the oil in a deep pot over a medium-high temperature. Add onion and garlic and stir-fry for 2-3 minutes or until translucent.

Now, add all remaining ingredients except shrimps. Stir well and bring it to a boil, or until thickened. Remove from the heat and transfer the mixture to a large baking sheet.

Spread the mixture evenly and put it in the oven. Bake for 20 minutes, then top with shrimps. Sprinkle some extra salt and pepper to taste if needed. Bake for another 5 minutes then remove from the oven. Let it cool for a while and serve.

Nutrition information per serving: Kcal: 252, Protein: 18.0g, Carbs: 32.0g, Fats: 5.7g

25. Orange Carrot Soup

Ingredients:

1 lb of carrots, shredded

5 large oranges, chopped

1 cup of chicken broth

3 oz of potatoes, peeled and chopped

2 small onions, chopped

1 garlic clove, minced

¼ cup of Greek yogurt

1 tsp of honey

1 tbsp of olive oil

½ tsp of ginger, minced

5 tbsp of lemon juice

½ tsp of salt

½ tsp of black pepper, ground

Preparation:

Combine lemon juice, mint, salt, and pepper in a mixing bowl. Mix well and set aside.

Preheat the oil in a large nonstick saucepan over a medium-high temperature. Add carrots, garlic, and onions and cook for about 1-2 minutes. Now, add all remaining ingredients except yogurt and bring it to a boil. Reduce the heat to low and cover with a lid. Cook for 15 minutes more and add the lemon mixture. Cook for 5 minutes more and remove from the heat. Stir in yogurt. You can add a few fresh orange chops before serving.

Nutrition information per serving: Kcal: 100, Protein: 2.9g, Carbs: 19.3g, Fats: 1.9g

26. Sunflower Smoothie

Ingredients:

1 large banana, chopped

1 medium-sized pear, cored and chopped

1 cup of Greek yogurt

¼ tsp of cumin

1 tbsp of honey

1 tbsp of sunflower seeds

Preparation:

Combine banana, pear, yogurt, cumin, and honey in a food processor. Blend until nicely smooth and transfer to a serving glasses. Top with sunflower seeds and refrigerate for 30 minutes before serving.

Nutrition information per serving: Kcal: 218, Protein: 11.5g, Carbs: 39.2g, Fats: 3.1g

27. Sweet Potato Oats

Ingredients:

1 cup of rolled oats

1 cup of sweet potatoes, peeled and chopped

¼ cup of dates, pitted and chopped

1 cup of almond milk

1 tsp of ginger, ground

½ tsp of cinnamon

1 tsp of liquid honey

¼ tsp of salt

Preparation:

Place sweet potatoes in a boiling water. Cook until fork-tender and remove from the heat. Drain well and transfer to a food processor. Blend until smooth and place it in a large bowl.

Stir in almond milk, oats, ginger, cinnamon, and honey. Sprinkle with a pinch of salt and mix well to combine.

Transfer the mixture to a medium skillet and cook for 10 minutes. Remove from the heat and stir in the dates.

Nutrition information per serving: Kcal: 597, Protein: 9.9g, Carbs: 75.9g, Fats: 31.6g

28. Cinnamon Strawberry Salad

Ingredients:

½ cup of strawberries, halved

½ cup of blueberries

½ cup of green grapes

1 medium-sized pear, cored and chopped

2 tbsp of lemon juice, freshly squeezed

1 cup of cream cheese

1 tsp of cinnamon, ground

¼ cup of almonds, roughly chopped

1 tbsp of chia seeds

Preparation:

Combine lemon juice, cream cheese, cinnamon, and chia seeds in a mixing bowl. Mix well to combine and set aside.

Combine fruits in a large salad bowl and toss once. Drizzle with dressing and give it a good stir. Top with almonds and refrigerate for 30 minutes before serving.

Nutrition information per serving: Kcal: 284, Protein: 6.2g, Carbs: 14.7g, Fats: 23.5g

29. Mushroom Meatballs

Ingredients:

1 lb of lean beef, minced

2 cups of chicken or beef stock

2 small onions, chopped

2 large eggs

1 cup of skim milk

1 cup of mushrooms

¼ cup of breadcrumbs

1 tbsp of all-purpose flour

1 tsp of vegetable seasoning mix

1 cup of sour cream

½ tsp of salt

¼ tsp of black pepper, ground

Preparation:

Whisk the eggs, breadcrumbs, and milk in a large mixing bowl. Add meat and squeeze with hand to combine.

Preheat a large nonstick skillet over a medium-high temperature. Shape the balls and place into the pan. Cook until browned. Add mushrooms, onions and chicken stock.reduce the heat to low and cover with a lid. Cook for about 25-30 minutes.

Meanwhile, combine flour, sour cream,salt, and pepper in a separate bowl. Stir well and pour the mixture into the skillet. Cook until the mixture thickened. Remove from the heat and serve warm.

Nutrition information per serving: Kcal: 226, Protein: 22.4g, Carbs: 8.0g, Fats: 11.2g

30. Grilled Salmon with Veggies

Ingredients:

2 lbs of salmon filets, skinless and boneless

1 cup of red wine vinegar

2 tbsp of olive oil

2 tbsp of maple syrup

2 garlic cloves, minced

1 cup of green beans, trimmed and chopped

1 cup of cauliflower, chopped

2 small carrots, chopped

½ tsp of salt

¼ tsp of black pepper, ground

Preparation:

Place green beans, cauliflower, and carrots in a pot of boiling water. Cook for 10 minutes, or until soften. Remove from the heat and set aside.

Preheat the oil in a large skillet over a medium-high temperature. Add vinegar, syrup, and garlic. Stir-fry for 1 minute and add meat. Bring it to a boil, then reduce the heat. Cover with a lid and cook for 5 minutes, stirring occasionaly.

Nutrition information per serving: Kcal: 284, Protein: 30.2g, Carbs: 9.1g, Fats: 14.1g

31. Turkey Carrot Salad

Ingredients:

1 lb of turkey breasts, skinless and boneless

5 oz of Romaine lettuce

3 large carrots, grated

¼ cup of Parmesan cheese, grated

5 tbsp of olive oil

1 tsp of Worcestershire sauce

1 tbsp of balsamic vinegar

1 garlic clove, minced

1 tbsp of lemon juice

½ tsp of salt

½ tsp of black pepper, ground

Preparation:

Combine oil, sauce, vinegar, garlic, lemon juice, salt, and pepper in a small bowl or a jar. Mix well to blend. Place the meat into a glass bowl and coat with marinade. Refrigerate for at least 1 hour.

Preheat a large nonstick frying pan over a medium-high temperature. Add meat and cook for 5 minutes on each side. Add carrots and cook for 2 more minutes. Remove from the heat and cut the into bite-sized pieces, or strips.

On a serving plate, make a fine layer of lettuce and top with meat and carrots. Sprinkle with grated cheese and some extra salt and pepper to taste.

Nutrition information per serving: Kcal: 340, Protein: 24.1g, Carbs: 12.4g, Fats: 22.2g

32. Mushroom Wraps

Ingredients:

1 lb of button mushrooms, finely chopped

1 cup of spring onions, finely chopped

1 cup of shallots, finely chopped

1 cup of frozen corn, thawed

2 tbsp of cilantro, chopped

½ tsp of red pepper, ground

2 garlic cloves, minced

1 tsp of ginger, grated

1 tsp of lime zest

½ cup of lime juice

½ cup of cream cheese

1 tsp of mint, finely chopped

½ tsp of salt

4 lettuce leaves

Preparation:

Mix together cream cheese, lime juice, lime zest, red pepper, garlic, and ginger in a medium bowl and set aside.

Preheat a large nonstick saucepan over a medium-high temperature. Add mushrooms, shallots, spring onions and 1 cup of water. Add cream mixture and cook for 5 minutes. Stir in corn, cilantro, and sprinkle with some salt and pepper to taste. Cook for another 2 minutes and then remove from the heat. Let it cool for a while.

Place lettuce leaves on the serving plates and spoon the mixture onto it. Wrap and secure with lid. Serve.

Nutrition information per serving: Kcal: 205, Protein: 8.8g, Carbs: 22.5g, Fats: 11.1g

33. Texas Spicey Spinach

Ingredients:

2 cups of black-eyed peas, pre-cooked

2 cups of fresh spinach, chopped

1 medium-sized tomato, diced

2 cups of corn, kernels removed

2 small onions, chopped

2 red bell pepper, chopped

2 garlic cloves, minced

1 small jalapeno pepper, chopped

For the dressing:

2 tbsp of balsamic vinegar

2 tbsp of olive oil

½ tsp of red pepper, ground

1 tsp of salt

¼ tsp of red pepper, ground

1 tsp of cumin, ground

Preparation:

Mix together all dressing ingredients and set aside to allow flavors to mingle.

Place the beans in a pot of boiling water and cook until soften. Remove from the heat and drain well. Transfer the beans in large bowl. Add remaining ingredients except the spinach and toss well.

Place a handful of spinach on a serving plate. Top with the previously made mixture. Drizzle all with dressing and sprinkle with extra salt if needed. Serve.

Nutrition information per serving: Kcal: 181, Protein: 7.1g, Carbs: 28.5g, Fats: 6.2g

34. Sweet Kale Smoothie

Ingredients:

2 cups of fresh kale, chopped

1 large banana, chopped

1 cup of almond milk

1medium-sized apple, cored and chopped

1 tbsp of honey

1 tbsp of walnuts

Preparation:

Combine all ingredients except walnuts in a food processor. Blend until finely smooth and transfer to a serving glasses. Top with almond and refrigerate for 1 hour before serving.

Nutrition information per serving: Kcal: 322, Protein: 4.5g, Carbs: 35.7g, Fats: 20.9g

35. Creamy Chicken

Ingredients:

12 oz of chicken breasts, skinless and boneless

1 tbsp of butter, melted

½ cup of cheddar cheese, crumbled

½ cup of cream cheese

2 tbsp of fresh parsley, finely chopped

1 tsp of Cayenne pepper, ground

1 tsp of salt

¼ tsp of black pepper, ground

Preparation:

Melt the butter in a large nonstick skillet over a medium-high temperature. Add chicken chops and cook for 10 minutes or until golden brown.

Stir in cream cheese, parsley, and cayenne pepper. Sprinkle with some salt and pepper and cook for 2 minutes. Remove from the heat and let it cool for a while.

Serve with rice, pasta or fresh veggies.

Nutrition information per serving: Kcal: 463, Protein: 40.6g, Carbs: 1.9g, Fats: 32.1g

36. Fennel with Oranges

Ingredients:

2 cups of fennel, trimmed and chopped

5 large oranges, chopped

3 cups of arugula, trimmed

2 cups of white beans, pre-cooked

2 tbsp of lemon juice

2 tbsp of balsamic vinegar

½ tsp of vegetable seasoning mix

¼ tsp of sweet pepper, ground

½ tsp of salt

¼ tsp black pepper, ground

Preparation:

Mix together lemon juice, vinegar, vegetable seasoning mix, sweet pepper, salt, and pepper in a mixing bowl. Set aside to allow flavors to meld.

Place beans in a pot of boiling water. Cook until soften and remove from the heat. Drain well and transfer to a large salad bowl. Add oranges, fennel, and arugula and toss well to combine.

Drizzle the dressing over the salad and serve immediately.

Nutrition information per serving: Kcal: 312, Protein: 17.9g, Carbs: 61.7g, Fats: 0.9g

37. Pumpkin Stew with Cumin Seeds

Ingredients:

1 lb of pumpkin, peeled and chopped

1 medium-sized onion, chopped

2 garlic cloves, minced

2 large carrots, sliced

2 celery stalks, chopped

2 tbsp of tomato paste

1 cup of spring onions, chopped

½ tsp of cumin seeds, toasted

4 cups of vegetable broth

1 tbsp of olive oil

½ tsp of salt

¼ tsp of black pepper, ground

Preparation:

Preheat the oil in a deep pot over a medium-high temperature. Add onions, garlic, and carrot and stir-fry for 3 minutes, or until translucent. Stir in about 2-3 tablespoons of water, cumin seeds, pumpkin chops, and tomato paste. Pour the vegetable broth and stir all well. Reduce the heat to low and cover with a lid. Simmer for 40 minutes, or until pumpkin is fork-tender.

Now, add celery, and cook for 5 minutes more. Remove from the heat and top with spring onions. Serve.

Nutrition information per serving: Kcal: 86, Protein: 3.8g, Carbs: 10.3g, Fats: 2.7g

38. Baked Maple Apple Crisps

Ingredients:

3 lbs of green apples, cored and sliced

1 tsp of cinnamon, ground

1 tsp of ginger, ground

2 tbsp of cornstarch

1 tsp of maple syrup

For the topping:

1 tsp of maple syrup

1 tbsp of honey

3 tbsp of butter

½ tsp of cinnamon, ground

2 tbsp of applesauce

1 tsp of vanilla extract

1 cup of rolled oats

½ tsp of salt

Preparation:

Preheat the oven to 375°F.

Combine apples, ginger, cornstarch, maple syrup, honey, and cinnamon in a large bowl. Stir well to coat the apples.

Mix together all topping ingredients in a large bowl. Stir well to combine.

Spread the apple mixture on a large baking sheet. Add another layer of topping mixture and put it in the oven. Bake for 15 minutes then reduce the temperature to 350°F. Bake until golden brown.

Nutrition information per serving: Kcal: 145, Protein: 1.7g, Carbs: 24.6g, Fats: 5.2g

39. Almond Muesli

Ingredients:

1 cup of rolled oats

2 tbsp of almonds, roughly chopped

½ cup of dates, pitted and chopped

½ tsp of cinnamon, ground

1 large banana, sliced

½ cup of almond milk

5 tbsp of coconut, toasted

Preparation:

Combine all ingredients except almonds in a large glass bowl. Toss well to combine and refrigerate for 15 minutes to soak. Top with almonds before serving.

Nutrition information per serving: Kcal: 559, Protein: 10.3g, Carbs: 83.6g, Fats: 24.5g

Juices

1.   Fennel Spinach Juice

Ingredients:

1 cup of fennel, chopped

1 cup of collard greens, torn

3 large green apples, cored

1 cup of fresh spinach, torn

Preparation:

Wash the fennel bulb and trim off the wilted outer layers. Cut into small chunks and fill the measuring cup. Reserve the rest in the refrigerator.

In a large colander, combine collard greens and spinach. Rinse thoroughly under cold running water and drain. Torn with hands and set aside.

Wash the apples and cut in half. Remove the core and cut into bite-sized pieces. Set aside.

Now, combine fennel, collard greens, spinach and apple in a juicer. Process until well juiced.

Transfer to a serving glass and refrigerate for 15 minutes

before serving.

Enjoy!

Nutritional information per serving: Kcal: 220, Protein: 5g, Carbs: 66.3g, Fats: 1.3g

2.   Cucumber Broccoli Juice

Ingredients:

1 cup of cucumber, sliced

2 cups of broccoli, chopped

1 cup of Brussels sprouts

1 teaspoon of olive oil

Preparation:

Wash the cucumber and cut into thin slices. Fill the measuring cup and reserve the rest for later. Set aside.

Wash the broccoli and trim off the outer layers. Cut into small pieces and set aside.

Wash the Brussels sprouts and trim off the outer wilted leaves. Cut in half and set aside.

Now, combine Cucumber, Broccoli and Brussels sprouts in a juicer and process until well juiced and add one teaspoon of olive oil before serving.

Serve immediately.

Enjoy!

Nutrition information per serving: Kcal: 74, Protein: 8.4g, Carbs: 21.8g, Fats: 1g

3.   Cauliflower Broccoli Juice

Ingredients:

1 cup of cauliflower, chopped

1 cup of fresh basil, torn

2 cups of broccoli, chopped

1 medium-sized red apple, cored

1 large lemon, peeled

Preparation:

Trim off the outer leaves of a cauliflower. Wash it and fill and cut into small pieces. Fill the measuring cup and reserve the rest in the refrigerator.

Wash the broccoli and chop into small pieces. Set aside.

Wash the apple and cut lengthwise in half. Remove the core and cut into bite-sized pieces. Set aside.

Peel the lemon and cut lengthwise in half. Set aside.

Now, combine cauliflower, basil, broccoli, apple and lemon in a juicer. Process until well juiced and transfer to a serving glass.

Add few ice cubes and serve immediately.

Enjoy!

Nutritional information per serving: Kcal: 156, Protein: 9g, Carbs: 46.4g, Fats: 1.5g

4.   Zucchini Basil Juice

Ingredients:

1 small zucchini, chopped

1 cup of mustard greens, chopped

2 cups of fresh basil, chopped

1 whole lime, peeled

1 whole cucumber, sliced

Preparation:

Peel the zucchini and cut into bite-sized pieces. Set aside.

Combine fresh basil and mustard greens in a large colander. Wash thoroughly under cold running water. Roughly chop it and soak in lukewarm water for 10 minutes.

Peel the lime and cut lengthwise in half. Set aside.

Wash the cucumber and cut into thin slices. Set aside.

Now, combine zucchini, basil, mustard greens, lime, and cucumber in a juicer and process until well juiced. Transfer to a serving glass and refrigerate for 10 minutes before serving.

Enjoy!

Nutritional information per serving: Kcal: 126, Protein: 7.5g, Carbs: 38.8g, Fats: 1.4g

5.   Cauliflower Avocado Juice

Ingredients:

5 cauliflower flowerets, chopped

1 cup of avocado, cubed

1 whole lime, peeled

1 whole leek, chopped

Preparation:

Wash the cauliflower flowerets thoroughly and chop into small pieces. Set aside.

Peel the avocado and cut in half. Remove the pit and cut into small cubes. Fill the measuring cup and reserve the rest in the refrigerator. Set aside.

Peel the lime and cut lengthwise in half. Set aside.

Wash the leek and cut into small pieces. Set aside.

Now, combine cauliflower, avocado, lime, and leek in a juicer and process until juiced. Transfer to a serving glass and refrigerate for 10 minutes before serving.

Enjoy!

Nutritional information per serving: Kcal: 268, Protein: 5.7g, Carbs: 32.4g, Fats: 22.5g

6.   Apple Kale Juice

Ingredients:

1 medium-sized red apple, cored

1 cup of cucumber, sliced

2 cups of fresh kale, chopped

1 cup of watercress, torn

1 cup of fresh parsley, torn

1 oz of water

Preparation:

Wash the cucumber and cut into thin slices. Fill the measuring cup and reserve the rest for later. Set aside.

Wash the apple and cut lengthwise in half. Remove the core and cut into bite-sized pieces. Set aside.

Wash the kale thoroughly under cold running water. Chop into small pieces and set aside.

Combine watercress and parsley in a colander. Rinse well under cold running water and torn with hands. Set aside.

Now, combine cucumber, apple, kale, watercress, and parsley in a juicer and process until juiced. Transfer to a serving glass and stir in the water. Add some ice before serving.

Enjoy!

Nutritional information per serving: Kcal: 150, Protein: 9.1g, Carbs: 40.8g, Fats: 2g

7. Carrots Orange Juice

Ingredients:

2 medium-sized carrots, sliced

2 cups of broccoli, chopped

1 large orange, peeled

1 whole lemon, peeled

1 small ginger knob, peeled

Preparation:

Wash and peel the carrot. Cut into thin slices and set aside.

Trim off the outer leaves of the broccoli. Wash it and cut into bite-sized pieces. Set aside.

Peel the orange and divide into wedges. Cut each wedge in half and set aside.

Peel the lemon and cut lengthwise in half. Set aside.

Peel the ginger knob and set aside.

Now, combine carrots, broccoli, orange, lemon, and, ginger knob in a juicer. Process until juiced.

Transfer to a serving glass and refrigerate for 15 minutes before serving.

Nutritional information per serving: Kcal: 162, Protein: 8.7g, Carbs: 51.8g, Fats: 1.4g

8.   Kale Broccoli Juice

Ingredients:

1 cup of kale, roughly chopped

2 cups of broccoli, chopped

1 small green apple, cored

1 medium-sized asparagus spears, trimmed

1 whole lemon, peeled

1 cup of fresh parsley, torn

Preparation:

Rinse the kale under cold running water. Slightly drain and torn with hands. Set aside.

Trim off the outer leaves of the broccoli. Wash it and cut into bite-sized pieces. Set aside.

Wash the apple and cut in half. Remove the core and cut into bite-sized pieces. Set aside.

Wash the asparagus and trim off the woody ends. Cut into small pieces and set aside.

Peel the lemon and cut lengthwise in half. Set aside.

Add parsley in a colander. Rinse well under cold running water and torn with hands. Set aside.

Now, combine kale, broccoli, apple, asparagus, lemon and parsley in a juicer. Process until juiced.

Transfer to a serving glass and refrigerate for 15 minutes before serving.

Nutritional information per serving: Kcal: 154, Protein: 11.1g, Carbs: 45.3g, Fats: 2.1g

9.   Zucchini Parsnip Juice

Ingredients:

1 cup of cucumber, sliced

1 small zucchini, chopped

1 cup of parsnip, sliced

1 medium-sized carrot, sliced

¼ tsp of ginger, ground

Preparation:

Wash the cucumber and cut into slices. Fill the measuring cup and reserve the rest for later.

Peel the zucchini and cut into bite-sized pieces. Set aside.

Wash and slightly peel the parsnip. Cut into thin slices and fill the measuring cup. Reserve the rest for later. Set aside.

Wash and peel the carrot. Cut into thin slices and set aside.

Now, combine cucumber, zucchini, parsnip and carrot in a juicer and process until juiced.

Transfer to a serving glass and stir in the ginger. Refrigerate for 10 minutes before serving.

Enjoy!

Nutritional information per serving: Kcal: 161, Protein: 7g, Carbs: 48.1g, Fats 1.8g

10.   Carrot Apple Juice

Ingredients:

2 large carrots, sliced

2 small green apples, cored

1 small zucchini, chopped

1 large lime, peeled

¼ tsp of ginger, ground

Preparation:

Wash and peel the carrots. Cut into thin slices and set aside.

Wash the apple and cut in half. Remove the core and cut into bite-sized pieces. Set aside.

Peel the zucchini and cut into thin slices. Set aside.

Peel the lime and cut lengthwise in half. Set aside.

Now, combine carrots, apples, zucchini and lime in a juicer. Process until well juiced. Transfer to a serving glass and stir in the ginger.

Enjoy!

Nutritional information per serving: Kcal: 161, Protein: 7g, Carbs: 48.1g, Fats: 1.8g

11. Raspberries Basil Juice

Ingredients:

2 medium-sized carrots, sliced

2 cups of raspberries

1 cup of fresh basil, torn

1 whole lemon, peeled

1 small Granny Smith's apple, cored

Preparation:

Wash and peel the carrots. Cut into thin slices and set aside.

Using a colander, rinse the raspberries under cold running water. Slightly drain and set aside.

Wash the basil thoroughly and torn with hands. Set aside.

Peel the lemon and cut lengthwise in half. Set aside.

Wash the apple and cut in half. Remove the core and cut into bite-sized pieces. Set aside.

Now, combine carrots, raspberries, basil, lemon and apple in a juicer and process until juiced.

Transfer to a serving glass and add few ice cubes.

Serve immediately.

Enjoy!

Nutritional information per serving: Kcal: 223, Protein: 7.3g, Carbs: 79.5g, Fats: 2.8g

12.   Raspberry Carrot Juice

Ingredients:

1 cup of raspberries

1 cup of blackberries

1 cup of blueberries

2 large carrots, peeled and chopped

1 large orange, wedged

1 tsp of fresh rosemary, finely chopped

Preparation:

Using a colander, wash the raspberries in under cold running water. Slightly drain and set aside.

Combine blackberries and blueberries in a colander. Rinse under cold running water and drain. Set aside.

Wash the carrots and peel them. Cut into small chunks and set aside.

Peel the orange and divide into wedges. Set aside.

Now, combine raspberries, blueberries, blackberries, carrots, orange and rosemary in a juicer and process until well juiced. Transfer to a serving glass.

Refrigerate for 10 minutes before serving.

Nutritional information per serving: Kcal: 246, Protein: 7.6g, Carbs: 85.4g, Fats: 2.5g

13.   Collard greens Carrot Juice

Ingredients:

2 cup of cucumber, sliced

2 cups of collard greens, torn

1 cup of fresh parsley, chopped

3 medium-sized carrots, sliced

1 tsp of fresh rosemary, finely chopped

Preparation:

Wash the cucumber and cut into thin slices. Fill the measuring cup and reserve the rest for later. Set aside.

Wash the collard greens thoroughly under cold running water. Place them in a bowl and add 2 cups of boiling water. Let it soak for 10 minutes. Slightly drain and set aside.

Rinse the parsley under cold running water and chop into small pieces.

Wash and peel the carrot. Cut into thin slices and set aside.

Now, combine cucumber, collard greens, parsley, carrots, and rosemary in a juicer and process until juiced.

Transfer to a serving glass and refrigerate for 10 minutes before serving.

Nutritional information per serving: Kcal: 94, Protein: 6.3g, Carbs: 29g, Fats: 1.4g

14.   Avocado Collard Greens Juice

Ingredients

1 cup of avocado, cubed

2 cups of collard greens, torn

1 small Granny Smith's apple, cored

1 cup of watercress, torn

1 tsp of fresh rosemary, finely chopped

Preparation:

Peel the avocado and cut in half. Remove the pit and cut into small cubes. Fill the measuring cup and reserve the rest in the refrigerator. Set aside.

Wash the collard greens thoroughly under cold running water. Place them in a bowl and add 2 cups of boiling water. Let it soak for 10 minutes. Slightly drain and set aside.

Wash the apple and cut in half. Remove the core and cut into bite-sized pieces. Set aside.

Wash the watercress and torn with hands. Set aside.

Now, combine avocado, collard greens, apples, watercress

and rosemary in a juicer.

Process until well juiced and transfer to a serving glass. Refrigerate for 10 minutes before serving.

Nutritional information per serving: Kcal: 389, Protein: 8.1g, Carbs: 43.5g, Fats: 34.4g

15.   Mixed Berry Juice

Ingredients:

1 cup of cranberries

1 cup of blackberries

1 cup of blueberries

1 large lime, peeled

1 large cucumber, chopped

1 cup of parsnip, sliced

Preparation:

Combine cranberries, blackberries and blueberries in a colander. Rinse under cold running water and drain. Set aside.

Peel the lime and cut lengthwise in half. Set aside.

Wash the cucumber and cut into small chunks. Set aside.

Wash and slightly peel the parsnip. Cut into thin slices and fill the measuring cup. Reserve the rest for later. Set aside.

Now, combine cranberries, blackberries, blueberries, cucumber, lime and parsnip in a juicer and process until juiced. Transfer to serving glasses and stir in the water.

Add some ice or refrigerate for 15 minutes before serving.

Nutritional information per serving: Kcal: 243, Protein: 7g, Carbs: 82.3g, Fats: 2g

16. Apple Cranberry Juice

Ingredients:

1 small Granny Smith's apple, chopped

1 cup of cranberries

1 cup of watercress, torn

½ cup of fresh spinach, torn

1 small ginger knob, peeled

Preparation:

Wash the apple and remove the core. Cut into bite-sized pieces and set aside.

Place the cranberries in a colander and rinse thoroughly. Slightly drain and set aside.

Wash watercress and spinach thoroughly under cold running water. Drain and torn with hands. Set aside.

Peel the ginger and set aside.

Now, combine apple, cranberries, watercress, spinach, and ginger in a juicer and process until well juiced. Transfer to a serving glass and stir in some water if you like. However, it is optional.

Refrigerate for 15 minutes before serving.

Enjoy!

Nutritional information per serving: Kcal: 249, Protein: 3.8g, Carbs: 86.1g, Fats: 0.9g

17.   Fennel Collard Green Juice

Ingredients:

1 cup of fennel, chopped

1 cup of collard greens, torn

1 large green apple, cored

A handful of spinach

1 teaspoon of olive oil

Preparation:

Wash the fennel bulb and trim off the wilted outer layers. Cut into small chunks and fill the measuring cup. Reserve the rest in the refrigerator.

In a large colander, combine collard greens and spinach. Rinse thoroughly under cold running water and drain. Torn with hands and set aside.

Wash the apple and cut in half. Remove the core and cut into bite-sized pieces. Set aside.

Now, combine fennel, collard greens, spinach, and apple in a juicer. Process until well juiced.

Transfer to a serving glass and add one teaspoon of olive

oil and refrigerate for 15 minutes before serving.

Enjoy!

Nutritional information per serving: Kcal: 122, Protein: 3.9g, Carbs: 37.4g, Fats: 0.9g

18. Avocado Kale Juice

Ingredients:

1 cup of fresh spinach, torn

1 cup of fresh kale, torn

1 cup of fresh parsley, torn

1 cup of cucumber, sliced

1 cup of avocado, chunked

¼ tsp of turmeric, ground

Preparation:

Combine spinach, kale, and parsley in a large colander. Rinse all under cold running water and slightly drain. Torn with hands and set aside.

Wash the cucumber and cut into thin slices. Set aside.

Peel the avocado and cut in half. Remove the pit and cut into small chunks. Fill the measuring cup and reserve the rest for later.

Now, combine spinach, kale, parsley, cucumber and avocado in a juicer and process until juiced. Transfer to a serving glass and stir in the turmeric.

Refrigerate for 10 minutes and serve.

Enjoy!

Nutritional information per serving: Kcal: 285, Protein: 17.3g, Carbs: 34.8g, Fats: 24.4g

19. Grapefruit Carrots Juice

Ingredients:

1 cup of raspberries

2 large oranges, wedged

2 large carrots, peeled and chopped

1 whole grapefruit, wedged

1 small ginger knob

Preparation:

Using a colander rinse raspberries under cold running water and drain. Set aside.

Peel the orange and divide into wedges. Cut each wedge in half and set aside.

Wash the carrots and peel them. Cut into small chunks and set aside.

Peel the grapefruit and divide into wedges. Cut each wedge in half and set aside.

Now, combine raspberries, orange, carrots, grapefruit and ginger in a juicer and process until well juiced. Transfer to a serving glass and stir in the coconut water.

Enjoy!

Nutritional information per serving: Kcal: 304, Protein: 8.2g, Carbs: 99g, Fats: 1.9g

20.   Orange Celery Juice

Ingredients:

2 small oranges, wedged

2 medium-sized celery stalks

1 small apple, cored

1 cup of raspberries

1 small ginger knob

Preparation:

Peel the orange and divide into wedges. Set aside.

Wash the celery and cut into bite-sized pieces. Set aside.

Wash the apple and cut in half. Remove the core and cut into bite-sized pieces. Set aside.

Using a colander wash the raspberries in under cold running water. Slightly drain and set aside.

Now, combine orange, celery, apple, raspberries and ginger in a juicer and process until well juiced. Transfer to a serving glass and add some crushed ice.

Serve immediately.

Enjoy!

Nutrition information per serving: Kcal: 185, Protein: 4.5g, Carbs: 60.3g, Fats: 1.4g

21.   Romaine lettuce Spinach Juice

Ingredients:

1 cup of fresh coriander, chopped

1 cup of fresh spinach, torn

1 cup of Romaine lettuce, shredded

1 whole cucumber, sliced

1 teaspoon of olive oil

Preparation:

Combine coriander, spinach, and lettuce in a large colander. Wash thoroughly under cold running water and slightly drain. Roughly chop all and set aside.

Wash the cucumber and cut into thin slices. Set aside.

Now, combine coriander, spinach, lettuce, and cucumber in a juicer and process until well juiced.

Transfer to a serving glass and add one teaspoon of olive oil before serving.

Serve immediately.

Enjoy!

Nutrition information per serving: Kcal: 85, Protein: 10.3g, Carbs: 23.9g, Fats: 1.8g

22.   Carrot Cucumber Juice

Ingredients:

4 medium-sized carrots, sliced

1 whole lime, peeled

2 cups of cucumber, sliced

1 small zucchini, chopped

1 medium-sized orange, wedged

1 tbsp of honey

Preparation:

Wash and peel the carrots. Cut into thin slices and set aside.

Peel the lime and cut lengthwise in half. Set aside.

Wash the cucumber and cut into thin slices. Fill the measuring cup and reserve the rest for later.

Peel the zucchini and cut lengthwise in half. Scrape out the seeds and wash it. Cut into small pieces and set aside.

Peel the orange and divide into wedges. Cut each wedge in half and set aside.

Now, combine carrots, lime, cucumber, zucchini and orange in a juicer and process until juiced.

Transfer to a serving glass and stir in the honey.

Add some ice before serving.

Enjoy!

Nutrition information per serving: Kcal: 161, Protein: 5.8g, Carbs: 49.9g, Fats: 1.2g

23.   Raspberries Oranges Juice

Ingredients:

4 large carrots, peeled and chopped

2 cups of raspberries

2 large oranges, wedged

¼ tsp of ginger, ground

Preparation:

Wash the carrots and peel them. Cut into small chunks and set aside.

Using a colander rinse the raspberries under cold running water and drain. Set aside.

Peel the oranges and divide into wedges. Set aside.

Now, combine carrots, raspberries and oranges in a juicer and process until well juiced. Transfer to a serving glass and stir in the ginger.

Refrigerate for 15 minutes before serving.

Enjoy!

Nutritional information per serving: Kcal: 274, Protein: 8.7g, Carbs: 96.3g, Fats: 2.6g

24.   Cauliflower Basil Juice

Ingredients:

2 cup of cauliflower, chopped

1 cup of fresh basil, torn

1 cup of beet greens, torn

1 cup of broccoli, chopped

1 large lemon, peeled

2 large oranges, wedged

1 medium-sized red apple, cored

Preparation:

Trim off the outer leaves of a cauliflower. Wash it and fill and cut into small pieces. Fill the measuring cup and reserve the rest in the refrigerator.

Combine basil and beet greens in a large colander. Rinse under cold running water and drain. Torn with hands and set aside.

Wash the broccoli and chop into small pieces. Set aside.

Peel the lemon and cut lengthwise in half. Set aside.

Peel the oranges and divide into wedges. Set aside.

Wash the apple and cut lengthwise in half. Remove the core and cut into bite-sized pieces. Set aside.

Now, combine cauliflower, basil, broccoli, beet greens, lemon, oranges and apple in a juicer. Process until well juiced and transfer to a serving glass.

Add few ice cubes and serve immediately.

Enjoy!

Nutritional information per serving: Kcal: 290, Protein: 13.1g, Carbs: 90.3g, Fats: 2g

25. Apple Brussels sprouts Juice

Ingredients:

1 medium-sized apple, cored

1 cup of Brussels sprouts

1 medium-sized carrot, chopped

1 whole lemon, peeled

2 large oranges, wedged

2 oz of water

Preparation:

Wash the apple and cut lengthwise in half. Remove the core and cut into bite-sized pieces. Set aside.

Wash the Brussels sprouts and trim off the outer wilted leaves. Cut in half and set aside.

Wash and peel the carrot. Cut into small chunks and set aside.

Peel the lemon and cut lengthwise in half. Set aside.

Peel the orange and divide into wedges. Cut each wedge in half and set aside.

Now, combine apple, Brussels sprouts, carrot, lemon and oranges in a juicer. Process until nicely juiced. Transfer to a serving glass.

Add some ice or refrigerate for 10 minutes before serving.

Enjoy!

Nutritional information per serving: Kcal: 367, Protein: 11.6g, Carbs: 113.8g, Fats: 2g

26. Zucchini Broccoli Juice

Ingredients:

1 small zucchini, chopped

1 cup of broccoli, chopped

1 cup of Brussels sprouts

1 cup of cucumber, sliced

1 small ginger slice, peeled

1 teaspoon of olive oil

Preparation:

Wash the broccoli and trim off the outer layers. Cut into small pieces and set aside.

Peel the zucchini and cut into bite-sized pieces. Set aside.

Wash the Brussels sprouts and trim off the outer wilted leaves. Cut in half and set aside.

Wash the cucumber and cut into thin slices. Fill the measuring cup and reserve the rest for later. Set aside.

Now, combine zucchini, broccoli, Brussels sprouts, cucumber and ginger in a juicer and process until well juiced.

Transfer to a serving glass and add one teaspoon of olive oil before serving.

Serve immediately.

Enjoy!

Nutrition information per serving: Kcal: 160, Protein: 15.3g, Carbs: 41.5g, Fats: 1.6g

27. Avocado Asparagus Juice

Ingredients:

1 cup of fresh asparagus, trimmed

1 cup of avocado, cubed

1 small Golden Delicious apple, cored

1 whole lime, peeled

1 cup of Swiss chard, torn

1 small ginger knob, peeled

Preparation:

Wash the asparagus and trim off the woody ends. Cut into bite-sized pieces and set aside.

Peel the avocado and cut lengthwise in half. Remove the pit and cut into small chunks. Set aside.

Wash the apple and remove the core. Cut into bite-sized pieces and set aside.

Peel the lime and cut lengthwise in half. Set aside.

Rinse the Swiss chard thoroughly under cold running water and slightly drain. Torn with hands and set aside.

Peel the ginger knob and cut into small pieces. Set aside.

Now, process asparagus, avocado, apple, lime, chard, and ginger in a juicer. Transfer to a serving glass and refrigerate for 15 minutes before serving.

Enjoy!

Nutritional information per serving: Kcal: 313, Protein: 7.2g, Carbs: 46.4g, Fats: 22.5g

28.   Avocado Swiss chard Juice

Ingredients:

1 cup of avocado, sliced

1 cup of Swiss chard, torn

2 medium-sized carrots

1 whole lime, peeled

1 cup of fennel, chopped

1 teaspoon of olive oil

Preparation:

Rinse the Swiss chard thoroughly under cold running water and slightly drain. Torn with hands and set aside.

Peel the avocado and cut lengthwise in half. Remove the pit and cut into thin slices. Fill the measuring cup and reserve the rest for later.

Wash and peel the carrots. Cut into small chunks and set aside.

Peel the lime and cut lengthwise in half. Set aside.

Wash the fennel bulb and trim off the wilted outer layers. Cut into small chunks and fill the measuring cup. Reserve the rest for some other juice.

Wash and peel the carrots. Cut into small chunks and set aside.

Now, combine avocado, Swiss chard, carrots, lime and fennel in a juicer and process until well juiced. Transfer to a serving glass and add one teaspoon of olive oil before serving.

Refrigerate for 15 minutes before serving.

Enjoy!

Nutritional information per serving: Kcal: 267, Protein: 6g, Carbs: 35.8g, Fats: 22.5g

29.   Avocado Zucchini Juice

Ingredients:

1 cup of avocado, chunked

1 small zucchini, chopped

1 whole lime, peeled

1 large orange, peeled

1 tsp of fresh mint, finely chopped

Preparation:

Peel the avocado and cut in half. Remove the pit and cut into chunks. Set aside.

Peel the zucchini and cut lengthwise in half. Scrape out the seeds and wash it. Cut into small pieces and set aside.

Peel the lime and cut lengthwise in half. Set aside.

Peel the orange and divide into wedges. Cut each wedge in half and set aside.

Now, combine avocado, zucchini, orange, lime, and mint in a juicer and process until juiced. Transfer to a serving glass and stir in the coconut water. Add some crushed ice and serve immediately.

Enjoy!

Nutritional information per serving: Kcal: 309, Protein: 5.8g, Carbs: 44.5g, Fats: 22.4g

30.   Avocado Fennel Juice

Ingredients:

1 cup of avocado, chunked

1 cup of fennel, chopped

1 small Granny Smith's apple, chopped

1 cup of cucumber, sliced

¼ tsp of ginger, ground

Preparation:

Peel the avocado and cut in half. Remove the pit and cut into small chunks. Fill the measuring cup and reserve the rest for later.

Wash the fennel bulb and trim off the wilted outer layers. Cut into small chunks and fill the measuring cup. Reserve the rest in the refrigerator.

Wash the apple and remove the core. Cut into bite-sized pieces and set aside.

Wash the cucumber and cut into thin slices. Fill the measuring cup and reserve the rest in the refrigerator. Set aside.

Now, combine avocado, fennel, apple, and cucumber in a juicer and process until juiced. Transfer to a serving glass and stir in the ginger.

Add some ice before serving.

Nutritional information per serving: Kcal: 286, Protein: 5g, Carbs: 40.3g, Fats: 21.9g

31.   Mustard Green Swiss Chard Juice

Ingredients:

2 cups of mustard greens, torn

2 cups of fresh spinach, torn

2 large carrots, sliced

2 cups of Swiss chard, torn

1 tsp of fresh rosemary, finely chopped

Preparation:

Wash mustard greens and spinach thoroughly under cold running water. Slightly drain and torn with hands. Set aside.

Wash the spinach thoroughly and slightly drain. Torn with hands and set aside.

Wash and peel the carrot. Cut into thin slices and set aside.

Rinse the Swiss chard thoroughly under cold running water and slightly drain. Torn with hands and set aside.

Now, combine mustard greens, spinach, carrot, Swiss chard and rosemary in a juicer and process until juiced.

Refrigerate for 15 minutes before serving.

Enjoy!

Nutritional information per serving: Kcal: 78, Protein: 7.5g, Carbs: 23.9g, Fats: 1.2g

32.   Pepper Celery Juice

Ingredients:

1 cup of fresh kale, torn

1 medium-sized celery stalk, chopped

1 cup of green peas

1 cup of fresh spinach, torn

¼ tsp of salt

Preparation:

Combine kale and spinach in a colander. Wash thoroughly under cold running water and slightly drain. Torn with hands and set aside.

Wash the celery stalk and cut into small pieces. Set aside.

Rinse the green peas using a colander. Place them in a bowl and soak in water for at least 30 minutes before using. You can also cook peas to soften. However, it's optional.

Now, combine kale, celery, peas and spinach in a juicer and process until juiced. Transfer to a serving glass and stir in the salt.

Serve immediately.

Enjoy!

Nutritional information per serving: Kcal: 166, Protein: 21g, Carbs: 41.5g, Fats: 2.6g

33.   Spinach Green Bean Juice

Ingredients:

1 cup of fresh spinach, chopped

1 cup of green beans, chopped

1 medium-sized Granny Smith's apple, cored

1 medium-sized celery stalk, cut into bite-sized pieces

1 teaspoon of olive oil

Preparation:

Wash the spinach thoroughly under cold running water. Chop into small pieces and fill the measuring cup. Reserve the rest for later.

Wash the green beans and chop into bite-sized pieces. Fill the measuring cup and reserve the rest for later.

Wash the apple and cut in half. Remove the core and cut into small chunks. Set aside.

Wash the celery and cut into bite-sized pieces. Set aside.

Now, combine spinach, green beans, apple and celery in a juicer and process until well juiced. Transfer to serving glass and add one teaspoon of olive oil before serving.

Add some ice before serving.

Enjoy!

Nutritional information per serving: Kcal: 140, Protein: 8.5g, Carbs: 37.3g, Fats: 1.4g

34.   Grapefruit Blueberries Juice

Ingredients:

1 whole grapefruit, wedged

1 cup of blueberries

1 small Golden Delicious apple, cored

¼ tsp of cinnamon, ground

Preparation:

Peel the grapefruit and divide into wedges. Cut each wedge in half and set aside.

Wash the blueberries using a colander. Slightly drain and set aside.

Wash the apple and cut in half. Remove the core and cut into bite-sized pieces. Set aside.

Now, combine grapefruit, blueberries, and apple in a juicer and process until juiced. Transfer to a serving glass and stir in the cinnamon.

Add some ice before serving and enjoy!

Nutritional information per serving: Kcal: 191, Protein: 2.1g, Carbs: 54.7g, Fats: 1g

35.   Avocado Cranberries Juice

Ingredients:

1 cup of avocado, cubed

1 whole lemon, peeled

1 cup of cranberries

1 cup of cucumber, sliced

1 small zucchini, chopped

1 cup of parsley, torn

Preparation:

Peel the avocado and cut into small cubes. Fill the measuring cup and reserve the rest in the refrigerator. Set aside.

Peel the lemon and cut lengthwise in half. Set aside.

Wash the cranberries and set aside.

Wash the cucumber and cut into slices. Fill the measuring cup and reserve the rest for later.

Peel the zucchini and cut into bite-sized pieces. Set aside.

Wash the parsley and torn with hands. Fill the measuring

cup and reserve the rest for later.

Now, combine avocado, cranberries, cucumber, parsley and zucchini in a juicer and process until juiced. Transfer to a serving glass and add some ice before serving.

Enjoy!

Nutritional information per serving: Kcal: 343, Protein: 8.6g, Carbs: 44.1g, Fats: 30.6g

36. Blackberry Grapefruit Juice

Ingredients:

1 cup of blackberries

1 whole grapefruit, wedged

1 medium-sized blood orange, peeled

1 whole lemon, peeled

2 medium-sized carrots, sliced

1 oz of water

Preparation:

Wash the blackberries thoroughly under cold water and slightly drain. Set aside.

Peel the grapefruit and divide into wedges. Cut each wedge in half and set aside.

Peel the orange and divide into wedges. Cut each wedge in half and set aside.

Peel the lemon and cut lengthwise in half. Set aside.

Wash and peel the carrots. Cut into thin slices and set aside.

Now, combine blackberries, grapefruit, orange, lemon and carrots in a juicer. Process until juiced and transfer to a serving glass.

Add some ice or refrigerate for a while before serving.

Enjoy!

Nutritional information per serving: Kcal: 216, Protein: 6.9g, Carbs: 72.5g, Fats: 1.6g

37. Granny Smith's apples Kale Juice

Ingredients:

1 cup of celery, chopped

2 small Granny Smith's apples, cored

1 cup of fresh kale, torn

1 whole lime, peeled

1 cup of broccoli, chopped

Preparation:

Wash the celery and chop into small pieces. Fill the measuring cup and set aside.

Wash the apple and cut in half. Remove the core and cut into bite-sized pieces. Set aside.

Wash the kale thoroughly under cold running water. Chop into small pieces and set aside.

Peel the lime and cut into small pieces. Set aside.

Wash the broccoli and cut into small pieces. Fill the measuring cup and reserve the rest in the refrigerator. Set aside.

Now, combine celery, apple, kale, lime and broccoli in a

juicer and process until juiced. Transfer to a serving glass and add some ice before serving.

Enjoy!

Nutritional information per serving: Kcal: 200, Protein: 7.58g, Carbs: 57.8g, Fats: 1.7g

38.   Broccoli Fennel Juice

Ingredients:

1 cup of broccoli, chopped

1 cup of fennel, chopped

1 cup of Brussels sprouts, halved

1 cup of watercress, torn

1 cup of cucumber, sliced

Preparation:

Wash the broccoli and cut into small pieces. Fill the measuring cup and reserve the rest in the refrigerator. Set aside.

Wash the fennel and trim off the outer leaves. Using a sharp paring knife, cut into small pieces and fill the measuring cup. Reserve the rest for later.

Wash the Brussels sprouts and trim off the outer layers. Cut in half and set aside.

Wash the watercress thoroughly under cold running water. Slightly drain and torn with hands. Set aside.

Wash the cucumber and cut into thin slices. Fill the

measuring cup and reserve the rest for later.

Now, combine broccoli, fennel, Brussels sprouts, watercress, and cucumber in a juicer and process until juiced. Transfer to a serving glass and refrigerate for 10 minutes before serving.

Enjoy!

Nutritional information per serving: Kcal: 72, Protein: 7.7g, Carbs: 22.6g, Fats: 0.8g

39.   Beet Green Carrot Juice

Ingredients:

1 cup of beet greens, torn

2 large carrots, sliced

1 whole grapefruit, wedged

1 medium-sized green apple, cored

1 medium-sized orange, peeled

¼ tsp of ginger, ground

Preparation:

Wash the beet greens thoroughly under cold running water. Drain and torn with hands. Set aside.

Wash the carrot and cut into thin slices. Set aside.

Peel the grapefruit and divide into wedges. Cut each wedge in half and set aside.

Peel the orange and divide into wedges. Cut each wedge in half and set aside.

Wash the apple and cut lengthwise in half. Remove the core and cut into bite-sized pieces. Set aside.

Now, combine beet greens, carrot, grapefruit, apple and orange in a juicer and process until juiced.

Transfer to a serving glass and stir in the ginger.

Serve cold.

Enjoy!

Nutritional information per serving: Kcal: 293, Protein: 7g, Carbs: 90.5g, Fats: 1.4g

40.   Cucumber Collard Greens Juice

Ingredients:

1 cup of cucumber, sliced

2 cups of collard greens, chopped

1 whole lime, peeled

1 cup of Swiss chard, chopped

1 large celery stalk, chopped

1 cup of fresh parsley, torn

1 oz of water

Preparation:

Combine collard greens and Swiss chard in a large colander. Wash it under running water and slightly drain. Chop into small pieces and set aside.

Wash the cucumber and cut into thin slices. Fill the measuring cup and reserve the rest in the refrigerator.

Peel the lime and cut lengthwise in half. Set aside.

Wash the celery and cut into small pieces. Set aside.

Add parsley in a colander. Rinse well under cold running

water and torn with hands. Set aside.

Now, combine collard greens, cucumber, lime, Swiss chard, and celery in a juicer and process until juiced. Transfer to a serving glass and stir in the water and salt. Refrigerate for 10 minutes before serving.

Enjoy!

Nutritional information per serving: Kcal: 40, Protein: 3.8g, Carbs: 12.7g, Fats: 0.7g

41.   Basil Avocado Juice

Ingredients:

1 cup of fresh basil, torn

1 cup of avocado, cubed

1 cup of fresh parsley, torn

1 cup of fresh spinach, chopped

1 cup of mustard greens, torn

¼ tsp of salt

Preparation:

Combine basil, parsley, and mustard greens in a colander. Rinse well under cold running water and slightly drain. Torn with hands and set aside.

Wash the spinach leaves and chop into small pieces. Fill the measuring cup and reserve the rest for later. Set aside.

Peel the avocado and cut in half. Remove the pit and cut into small cubes. Fill the measuring cup and reserve the rest in the refrigerator. Set aside.

Now, combine basil, parsley, mustard greens, spinach and avocado in a juicer and process until well juiced. Transfer to a serving glass and stir in the reserved tomato juice and salt.

Serve cold.

Enjoy!

Nutrition information per serving: Kcal: 64, Protein: 10.9g, Carbs: 17.9g, Fats: 1.8g

42.   Blueberry Grapefruit Juice

Ingredients:

2 cups of blueberries

1 small ginger knob, peeled and chopped

1 medium-sized blood orange, peeled

1 whole grapefruit, wedged

Preparation:

Place the blueberries in a colander. Wash thoroughly under cold running water and drain. Fill the measuring cups and reserve the rest in the freezer.

Peel the ginger and cut into small pieces. Set aside.

Peel the orange and divide into wedges. Cut each wedge in half and set aside.

Peel the grapefruit and divide into wedges. Cut each wedge in half and set aside.

Now, combine blueberries, ginger, orange, and grapefruit in a juicer and process until juiced.

Transfer to a serving glass and add few ice cubes before serving.

Enjoy!

Nutritional information per serving: Kcal: 282, Protein: 5.4g, Carbs: 85.5g, Fats: 1.5g

43.   Romaine lettuce Grapefruit Juice

Ingredients:

1 whole grapefruit, wedged

1 cup of Romaine lettuce, shredded

2 medium-sized carrots, sliced

1 cup of fresh mint, chopped

1 whole lime, peeled

Preparation:

Peel the grapefruit and divide into wedges. Cut each wedge in half and set aside.

Wash the lettuce thoroughly under cold running water. Shred it and fill the measuring cup. Reserve the rest for later.

Wash and peel the carrots. Cut into thin slices and set aside.

Wash the mint and then place it in a medium bowl. Add one cup of hot water and let it soak for 10 minutes. Slightly drain and set aside.

Peel the lime and cut lengthwise in half. Set aside.

Now, combine grapefruit, lettuce, carrots, mint, and lime in a juicer and process until juiced. Transfer to a serving glass and add some crushed ice before serving.

Enjoy!

Nutritional information per serving: Kcal: 147, Protein: 4.7g, Carbs: 46.8g, Fats: 1.1g

44.   Basil Broccoli Juice

Ingredients:

2 cups of cauliflower, chopped

1 cup of fresh basil, torn

1 cup of Swiss chard, torn

1 cup of broccoli, chopped

1 cup of beet greens, torn

1 large lemon, peeled

1 medium-sized green apple, cored

Preparation:

Trim off the outer leaves of a cauliflower. Wash it and fill and cut into small pieces. Fill the measuring cup and reserve the rest in the refrigerator.

Combine basil and beet greens in a large colander. Rinse under cold running water and drain. Torn with hands and set aside.

Rinse the Swiss chard thoroughly under cold running water and slightly drain. Torn with hands and set aside.

Wash the broccoli and chop into small pieces. Set aside.

Peel the lemon and cut lengthwise in half. Set aside.

Wash the apple and cut lengthwise in half. Remove the core and cut into bite-sized pieces. Set aside.

Now, combine cauliflower, basil, broccoli, beet greens, lemon, apple and Swiss chard in a juicer. Process until well juiced and transfer to a serving glass.

Add few ice cubes and serve immediately.

Enjoy!

Nutritional information per serving: Kcal: 138, Protein: 7.4g, Carbs: 41.4g, Fats: 1.3g

45.   Brussels Sprouts Kale Juice

Ingredients:

2 cups of Brussels sprouts, halved

1 medium-sized Granny Smith's apple, cored

1 cup of fresh mint, torn

1 cup of fresh kale, torn

1 whole lime, peeled

1 cup of broccoli, chopped

1 oz of water

Preparation:

Wash the Brussels sprouts and trim off the outer leaves. Cut in half and fill the measuring cup. Reserve the rest for later.

Wash the apple and cut in half. Remove the core and cut into bite-sized pieces. Set aside.

Combine mint and kale in a large colander and rinse under cold running water. Slightly drain and torn with hands. Set aside.

Peel the lime and cut lengthwise in half. Set aside.

Wash the broccoli and chop into small pieces. Set aside.

Now, combine Brussels sprouts, apple, mint, kale, lime and broccoli in a juicer and process until juiced. Transfer to a serving glass and stir in the water.

Refrigerate for 10 minutes before serving.

Enjoy!

Nutritional information per serving: Kcal: 171, Protein: 14g, Carbs: 74.4, Fats: 2.2g

46. Carrot Parsnip Juice

Ingredients:

2 medium-sized carrots, sliced

2 cups of parsnip, sliced

1 cup of cucumber, sliced

1 cup of watercress, torn

1 whole lemon, peeled

1 small ginger knob, peeled

1 tbsp of honey

Preparation:

Wash and peel the parsnips and carrots. Cut into thin slices and set aside.

Peel the cucumber and chop into chunks. Fill the measuring cup and reserve the rest for later.

Rinse the watercress under cold running water and slightly drain. Torn with hands and set aside.

Peel the lemon and cut lengthwise in half. Set aside.

Peel the ginger knob and cut into small pieces. Set aside.

Now, combine parsnip, carrot, cucumber, watercress, lemon, and ginger in a juicer and process until well juiced.

Transfer to a serving glass and stir in the honey.

Enjoy!

Nutritional information per serving: Kcal: 210, Protein: 6.2g, Carbs: 68.3g, Fats: 1.4g

47.   Fennel Mustard greens Juice

Ingredients:

1 cup of fennel, chopped

2 cups of mustard greens, torn

1 large leek, chopped

1 cup of fresh mint, torn

1 large green apple, cored

A handful of spinach

1 tbsp of liquid honey

Preparation:

Wash mustard greens and spinach thoroughly under cold running water. Slightly drain and torn with hands. Set aside

Wash the fennel bulb and trim off the wilted outer layers. Cut into small chunks and fill the measuring cup. Reserve the rest in the refrigerator.

Wash the leek and cut into bite-sized pieces. Set aside.

Wash the apple and cut in half. Remove the core and cut into bite-sized pieces. Set aside.

Now, combine fennel, mustard greens, mint, spinach, leek, and apple in a juicer. Process until well juiced.

Transfer to a serving glass and refrigerate for 15 minutes before serving.

Nutritional information per serving: Kcal: 180, Protein: 6.2g, Carbs: 53.7g, Fats: 1.4g

48. Kale Mustard Green Juice

Ingredients:

2 medium-sized green apples, cored

1 cup of cucumber, sliced

2 cups of fresh kale, chopped

1 cup of mustard greens, torn

1 cup of fresh spinach, torn

1 large carrot, sliced

1 tsp of fresh rosemary, finely chopped

Preparation:

Wash the apples and cut lengthwise in half. Remove the core and cut into bite-sized pieces. Set aside.

Wash the cucumber and cut into thin slices. Fill the measuring cup and reserve the rest for later. Set aside.

Wash the kale thoroughly under cold running water. Chop into small pieces and set aside.

Wash mustard greens and spinach thoroughly under cold running water. Slightly drain and torn with hands. Set aside.

Wash and peel the carrot. Cut into thin slices and set aside.

Now, combine apples, mustard greens, spinach, carrot and rosemary in a juicer and process until juiced.

Transfer to a serving glass and refrigerate for 15 minutes before serving.

Enjoy!

Nutritional information per serving: Kcal: 250, Protein: 11g, Carbs: 71.5g, Fats: 2.5g

ADDITIONAL TITLES FROM THIS AUTHOR

70 Effective Meal Recipes to Prevent and Solve Being Overweight: Burn Fat Fast by Using Proper Dieting and Smart Nutrition

By

Joe Correa CSN

48 Acne Solving Meal Recipes: The Fast and Natural Path to Fixing Your Acne Problems in Less Than 10 Days!

By

Joe Correa CSN

41 Alzheimer's Preventing Meal Recipes: Reduce or Eliminate Your Alzheimer's Condition in 30 Days or Less!

By

Joe Correa CSN

70 Effective Breast Cancer Meal Recipes: Prevent and Fight Breast Cancer with Smart Nutrition and Powerful Foods

By

Joe Correa CSN

www.ingramcontent.com/pod-product-compliance
Lightning Source LLC
Chambersburg PA
CBHW030250030426
42336CB00009B/319